From Paris With Love

A Personal and Supportive Guide to Breast Cancer

PRISCILLA LALISSE-JESPERSEN

Dedicated to my husband and children, who never gave up on me.

To my amazing oncologist, Dr. F. You have made all the difference.

I also dedicate this to all the women who are fighting breast cancer and in memory of all those who have died because of it.

And last but not least, to Stuart Scott, the American sportscaster who died of cancer in 2015, but not before teaching me that no matter what happens, I've already won.

Important Note to the Reader

The information found in this book is based on my personal experience as a breast cancer survivor. My journey started in Paris but ended so very far away—culturally, nationally and spiritually. Here is my story about breast cancer as a Black woman, a writer, a Christian, a mother, and a wife, while I endured painful and invasive treatments for my diagnosis, which I didn't always understand and which were often made more difficult by the way people saw me as a person of color.

Part memoir and part practical guide, this book is also influenced by the many conversations I have had with fellow survivors in which I have tried to provide all the advice I could think of for their own journeys. My goal? To make the fight against breast cancer just a little bit easier. As a writer by profession, I knew that I had to write a book about breast cancer, and many times when talking to another survivor I wished I had already completed the book so that people would have something in hand.

However, this book was so hard to write! I began in 2014 when I was diagnosed, but it took much longer than I anticipated to finish it. I had to put it aside for a while, partly because I found it difficult to revisit this period in my life. Yet, I never would have been satisfied if I hadn't seen it through. Finally, I have something I can share with other survivors (and caretakers). This book is my wish realized.

As much as I hope that the observations and insights contained in these pages will be useful, I must emphasize that they do not replace the guidance of your medical team. Everyone's diagnosis and experiences are different, so please remember that. Still, I hope you will find something helpful and reassuring in this book. If there is even the slightest thing that makes your life easier during this challenging time, then I feel I will have succeeded.

From Paris With Love

A Personal and Supportive Guide to Breast Cancer

CHAPTER 1

First Mammogram Ever

First. Mammogram. Ever.

That's how my breast cancer journey began

I had been living in Paris, France, for over 15 years and I was moving back to the United States, where I had gotten a good job and was excited about my family's new beginning there. Paris had been a dream. It was a great place to live and I had truly enjoyed being there, but I was eager to begin a new career back home.

While I was preparing for the move, I found a doctor's order for a mammogram. It was dated July 2013 and I had gotten it at my six-week checkup after my youngest child was born.

I had put off having a mammogram. I had made appointments, but I had always cancelled them for one reason or another: work, kids, and other commitments. *Life.* It is not that I thought mammograms were unimportant. My own mother had come face to face with Stage 0 breast cancer in 2006. However, this time, since I was moving, and I didn't know when or where I would be able to have a mammogram, I decided that I would try to keep the appointment.

But I almost didn't.

My mammogram was scheduled on May 12, the day before I was to fly to America. I thought I'd have to cancel it, but after work was delayed a couple of weeks, I was able to keep the appointment. Even so, I almost didn't go because I had so very many things to do in preparation for my big move back home.

I had no idea that that mammogram would change my life forever.

Chapter 2

My Doctor's Visit: May 12, 2014

I had so many things on my mind with my international move. A move is never easy, and the leap from one country and culture to another is ten times harder. I had three children to manage as well. School records, medical records, last-minute packing, telephone calls, you name it. As I was going to America ahead of my husband and the kids (for work-related training), it added to the stress and logistics. For me, the mammogram was just another administrative headache and one I'd rather put off. It was another thing to cross off my to-do list.

I arrived early in the morning for my appointment at a clinic at La Défense, a major business district of the Paris metropolitan area. I hoped that the staff would get me in and out quickly because I had many more errands to run.

When the technician finally called me back, I was relieved. He asked me to take off everything from my waist up, definitely not the most comfortable situation to be in. It was not the first time I had been examined by a male. In France, when it comes to medical exams, it sometimes seems there is no such thing as privacy. You do not get the little blue gowns that you need to leave open in the front or the back. The doctor's office and the exam room are often one and the same.

Nevertheless, I had a problem removing my bra and stepped out of the changing room with it still on. The technician looked at me with a slight smile and said, "You'll have to take off your bra, too."

Crap.

After finally getting my bra off, I felt a little awkward coming out of the changing room, with nothing to cover myself up save my arms. Luckily, the technician was going out of his way to distract me from the fact that he was lifting my breasts and placing them in the machine to be squeezed. He spoke about his upcoming trip to New York, and how excited he was. His enthusiasm was contagious, and my mind slipped off to plan my own little NYC escapade, as I would soon be living in Baltimore. The conversation relaxed me and made me forget that I was topless in front of a stranger.

Afterwards, I sat in the waiting room while he read the results. A few minutes later he came out and said he needed to follow up with an ultrasound. I was not worried at this point because he had already told me at the beginning of the mammogram that this was a possibility. So, for me, it was procedural.

A doctor then came in to speak to me. His name was Dr. K. and he spoke in perfect English. I did not know then that Dr. K. and his technician would be responsible for finding the cancerous tumors that threatened my life.

He performed the ultrasound and explained what he was doing and why. This was a different experience for me because many times French doctors just go right in and do their thing and get out. They don't talk, they don't explain, and you are left to go home and look on the internet to find out what just happened.

Dr. K. was different, however. "You see that?" he asked, pointing to the screen. "That's suspicious." I could not decipher a thing. The only thing I saw were gray images.

"What do you mean by suspicious?" I asked.

"Actually, there are two suspicious places, but I am mostly concerned with the larger one. If you put your fingers here, you can feel it."

And so, I did, and there it was, a large hard "thing" inside my left breast. I call it a thing because it did not feel like a lump. Remember when people talk about self-exams, they always say, "I felt a lump." Well, for me, it didn't feel circular or lumpish. It just felt large, and hard.

I had had no idea it was even there, before that moment.

"I need to perform a biopsy," Dr. K. said with a concerned expression. "Can you come back next week?"

"Actually, no, Doctor. I am going to the United States tomorrow."

"Tomorrow?"

"Yes, tomorrow."

"Would you like to do the biopsy there? Wait, let me see if we can fit you in this afternoon. Could you come then?"

"Yes, please fit me in if you can."

Now at this point I was a little bit concerned but still not in panic mode. I should have been because most of the time French doctors had not fit me in, anywhere. It can take days just to get your doctor on the phone, if ever. There are lots of walls, procedures, *c'est comme ca,* things. It's just not done. But here I was with a French doctor slightly urging me to be biopsied. Today.

Yet, still my brain said this: It is my first mammogram. Do they have a baseline? Nope, they don't. They have no point of reference here. Maybe I was like one of my friends who had told me that she had dense breasts. Other friends had fibroids. Any and all of this, but the thought of me actually having cancer was not even entertained.

I went back in the afternoon and had the biopsy. Dr. K. seemed happy with the sample he took. He was diligent and sympathetic. He was adequately concerned yet restrained. He wished me a *bon voyage* and told me that I would have the results in ten days. I left the office and went back home to finish packing.

Ten days, I thought. That's a long time to receive good news, but that's okay. I had an international move ahead of me and a lot on my plate. I would be extremely busy, and the time would fly by. I would get the results and the biopsy would be negative and this would all be behind me.

I sent an email to friends and family that briefly mentioned the mammogram and biopsy, but I was more interested in and excited by the fact that I had had a new article published in *The Washington Post* the day before, in honor of Mother's Day. My piece was entitled: "Not my mother's world: Living my mother's dream an ocean away". It was one of my favorite pieces because my mother is definitely a profile in courage. She raised five children while working and going to school full-time at one point. The piece had been well received so far. I had become a freelance writer for *The Washington Post* in July of 2013. It was a dream come true for me, and I loved it. I was happy and pleased with my article, and as I said, extremely busy with the move. So, I did not allow myself to get caught up in the whole suspicious mammogram thing.

Little did I know.

Practical Advice for Mammograms

1. First, never put off your mammograms. If you haven't had a mammogram this year, or ever—make your appointment ASAP.
2. Find a reputable facility and make an appointment. (If you can go to the same place each year, it will make it easier to track your results.)
3. Don't be afraid to have it. I've heard a lot of women say that the reason they don't have mammograms is because they're scared. The procedure can be unpleasant, stressful, and even painful for some. It's normal to feel trepidation, but don't let it overwhelm you. Just think of your health.
4. Relax before, during and after you have the mammogram.
5. It's okay that it's uncomfortable. Trust me, the discomfort is worth it, *especially* if it will help avoid aggressive treatments such as chemotherapy, radiation and surgery.
6. If your insurance allows, try to have the 3D mammogram. Studies show that 3D mammograms have found more cancers than the traditional 2D mammograms. The 3D mammogram also reduces the number of false positives. If you are in a lot of pain, tell the person administering your test. Also, let them know if you've noticed anything different about your breasts.
7. Remember that you are doing this for your health.
8. Be sure to have your exam yearly.

Chapter 3
What Will Be, Will Be

I hate it that hindsight is always 20/20.

After I left the doctor's office at La Défense, I continued running my errands. My mind just could not comprehend that I, in the middle of a transatlantic move, would have breast cancer. Absolutely not. Because if I had, I probably wouldn't have left France at all. If I had asked and pressed the doctor to tell me the odds of my having cancer, and had he given me those odds with any certainty, I suppose I would have stayed. The timing didn't help, either. I was flying out of Charles de Gaulle the next day. I had no time to think, to analyze and contemplate what was happening. And I wasn't going to get myself worked up for what I thought would be nothing.

But of course, that nothing was something—and what a big something it was.

Two weeks later, I had started my new job and was going through training. Everything was going well. My husband and kids were still in Paris but would be joining me in another week. It was at that time that I thought, "Hey, isn't it time to get those results?"

It was.

I called my doctor's office in Paris, the one who had performed the biopsy. It was a strange conversation. He led me to believe there was some cause for concern. He may even have told me I had breast cancer; I'm honestly not sure—but he didn't want to go into any real details over the phone. He referred me to my OB/GYN, who had given me the script to have the mammogram in the first place. My mind couldn't quite comprehend it. I needed more information, so I sat down on the freshly cleaned brown carpet of our newly acquired apartment in Baltimore and speedily dialed up my other doctor.

I'll never ever forget that conversation. Ever.

"Hello, Madame Jespersen, I'm glad you called. I need to see you in my office right away."

"I'm sorry, Dr. P., but I'm in America and I'm not returning to France any time soon," I said, suddenly rethinking it. "But I talked to Dr. K. and he told me about a potential cancer?"

"Madame Jespersen, yes. Yes, there was something in the results. That's why I wanted to see you. Can your husband come to my office today?"

"Yes, I'm sure he can."

"I'll wait for him, and then call you back."

"OK, Dr. P. Thank you!"

And then I hung up the phone and screamed.

~

A few hours later, my husband called me and confirmed what I already knew: I had breast cancer, and that was it. He didn't panic, but my brain was going a million miles a minute. My new job, my training, my children—my baby was only a year old, for crying out loud. My parents. My poor husband. My siblings. My friend. ME!

Yet, it was true. There was nothing I could do but find out *what* to do. Dr. P. called me back as promised and we discussed the next steps. Either I could come back to Paris and he'd get me started with treatment, or I could stay in Baltimore. When he asked what hospital was closest to me, I told him Johns Hopkins and that sealed the deal. He told me that I would be in good hands—that it was one of the best hospitals in the world. And it is. I would recommend it to anyone. When the doctors and nurses learned of my unique situation—of having been diagnosed in France—they did everything possible to ensure that all the bases were covered when it came to treating me. Because I'd had my initial mammogram, ultrasound and biopsy in France, everything was in French, of course. My doctors and the labs in Paris were more than happy to share these results with my American doctors, but in the end, it was decided that everything should be repeated. So, on my 46th birthday I found myself at the hospital having another mammogram, ultrasound, and biopsy.

By this time my husband and the kids had joined me from France, and that certainly made things a little bit easier. The results were unfortunately the same and would lead me on to further testing: two MRIs and a PET/CT Scan. I didn't have any trouble with the PET/CT Scan, which is an imaging test used with a radioactive drug to reveal how the tissues and organs in the body are functioning. On the other hand, the MRI, which also provides detailed pictures of the inside of your body, was pretty challenging. I don't consider myself claustrophobic, but during those moments in that darkened space where dark thoughts came so easily, I almost lost it. Lying there listening to the clicks of the machine, I understood why my grandmother hated MRIs so much. She called it the "chicken-breast" machine, although I am not sure why. But it had to be done, and there was no way that I was going to move or mess it up and have to start all over again. And so, I got through it.

CHAPTER 4

Handling Bad News

I was slightly out of breath when I got off the elevator at the Johns Hopkins Sidney Kimmel Cancer Center in downtown Baltimore. A week or so had passed since the scans and now it was time to learn the results and what they meant in terms of my diagnosis.

It had been tricky parking the car and getting to the exact place I needed to be. Wiping my forehead with a napkin I'd snagged from my bag, I checked in at a yellow kiosk manned by an elderly black gentleman whose name tag read "Billy."

"You can have a seat now, Miss," he said, pointing to the adjoining waiting room. Glancing around me, I headed that way, tiptoeing across the floor, trying not to make eye contact with the sea of bald heads who surrounded me.

My head would soon be bald, too, but I didn't want to think about it today.

Most of the patients passing time in the waiting room were wrinkly. They wore platform shoes and hearing aids. Some were white, some were black, and some were yellow and brown. Cancer is diverse, alright.

Some leaned on supporters, and some were alone, like me. I didn't mind. I wanted my husband, who was now in Baltimore, to stay back at our new apartment and keep our children busy. They didn't need to be in this gray room that smelled like sweat and antiseptic.

A nurse called me through yellow automatic doors and checked my vitals before placing me in a tiny room filled with medical diagrams. I'd just read about the lymphatic system when a 60-something-year-old doctor with thinning gray hair and gray eyes walked in. He was also wearing a gray sweater, tan Dockers, and sturdy brown shoes.

"Hello, I am Dr. F.," he said, with an outstretched hand and a small smile.

I rose to my feet and shook his hand. "Hi. Pleased to meet you, Doctor."

He pulled up a chair while pointing for me to take mine again.

I did and took out my notepad, ready to find out if I had Stage 1 or Stage 2 breast cancer and what that would entail. Placing my notepad in my lap and crossing my ankles, I took a deep breath, and waited.

"We received all your scans, the PET and MRIs. We've studied them carefully."

I continued holding my breath and watched him as he referred to something on the computer in front of him.

"Initially, we thought that your breast cancer was an earlier stage..."

I sat up straighter and prepared to write.

"However, we now know that it is a Stage 3."

Stunned, I cleared my throat. Perhaps I had misheard.

"Aren't there only 4 stages to breast cancer?" I asked, a tremor building in my voice.

"Yes. And then those 4 stages are divided into subcategories, which are a, b, and c based on tumor size and lymph nodes."

I slid forward to the end of my seat and uncrossed my ankles. "What is my exact stage, then?"

"Based on what we've seen, it's a Stage 3c."

"So, you are telling me that I'm almost a Stage 4?"

"Yes, I'm afraid so," he said, clasping his hands together on his swirly stool and staring at me.

"We are going to...of which that...your death..." he started again, but I lost track of his words.

Am I going to die? Am I going to die? Oh, Lord, am I going to die?

That's all I heard, my own voice over and over asking if I were going to die. I missed the part about needing 26 rounds of chemotherapy. I missed the part about needing six weeks of radiation. I didn't hear him say that it wasn't Stage 4 yet and that they would do their best. I just heard, *Am I going to die? Oh, Lord, am I going to die*? And that kept playing through my head like an old broken cassette tape until Dr. F. stood up and proffered his hand and said his nurse navigator would be in touch with me.

I stumbled out of the examination room, through the swoosh of the automatic doors, and passed the bald heads once again and made it to the garage. I put the Honda in drive and fumbled through my purse to pay the parking.

But the cassette tape wouldn't turn off. *Am I going to die? Oh, Lord, am I going to die*?

It sang on and on until the tears I had been withholding for the past 30 minutes escaped and flooded my face like that torrential rain I'd endured in South Korea once. What was it called? Monsoon rain?

The sun was high in the sky, but I could barely see the interstate. Cars whished by me. A man driving a transfer truck nearly ran me off the road and angrily blew his horn at me. Another man wearing what could have been a Jheri curl and driving a red caddy rolled down his window, took out his cigarette and glared at me.

I didn't care. I could barely see them. My body violently shook all over. I briefly closed my eyes to focus. I had to get home to my husband and kids and tell them that momma was much sicker than we thought.

I pressed my sandaled foot harder onto the gas pedal as I willed that cassette tape to stop torturing me, but all I heard all the way home was, "*Am I going to die? Oh, Lord, am I going to die?*"

Practical Advice for Handling a Diagnosis

1. When you're waiting for diagnosis, it's a crazy time. Your mind is reeling and you're anxious. That is normal. So, while you're waiting, just take it easy and engage in activities that will help you remain as calm as possible. Try to engage in activities that will help take your mind off the pending news, such as reading, exercising, knitting, or cooking, for example. Call up your friends and family. Read your Bible, or take solace in the Koran, Hebrew Bible, or the Tripitaka. Practice yoga. Meditate. *Breathe.*
2. Don't engage in *self-diagnosing through the internet.* Easier said than done, right? You'll be tempted to get right onto Google and find out your diagnosis, stage, treatment options, and life expectancy. Avoid it as best you can. I won't tell you it's easy—I attempted it at first. It is more harmful than helpful, trust me. Wait for your doctors to give you a professional diagnosis.
3. If possible, don't go to appointments by yourself. My sister accompanied me to my first appointment with my breast surgeon. To say that it helped tremendously is an understatement. Looking back on it now, I should not have gone alone to that first appointment with my oncologist. Handling devastating, surprising, bad news is much easier when you have someone you can lean on. And drive for you afterwards! Ask your oncologist questions and write down the answers. Some of the questions I asked were:
    - What is my exact diagnosis?
    - What stage of breast cancer do I have?

- Has the cancer metastasized?
- What exactly will my treatment entail?
- How frequent will my treatments be?
- What are the side effects of the treatment?
- Will my treatments affect my daily life?
- Can I still work?
- Will I be able to take care of my children?
- Do I need genetic testing?

4. You will be shaken. You will be shocked. You will be dazed at some point in all of this. But don't worry; that is normal in this situation. The most important thing is to get your diagnosis and then go forward with a plan. Try not to let yourself become crippled with fear.
5. Don't compare your diagnosis to someone else's. Every single case is different. I repeat, **every single case is different!** Learning this at the very beginning, and keeping it in mind throughout your journey, will help you in many ways.
6. Whether or not to tell your friends about your diagnosis is up to you! I have known people who only wanted their immediate family to know and I've known people who wanted the world to know. I suppose I was closer to the latter. It's not that I wanted the entire world to know, but I did want my friends and family to know. I made the right decision because the love, light and support that I received from people all around the world (I have friends scattered about the globe) was extremely helpful. I received so much love and encouragement. It was amazing. I still think about it to this day—how people went out of their way to cheer me up and make me smile during these difficult days. But that's me. You must make the right decision for *yourself.* Do what is most comfortable for you.

7. Tell your children. If I regret anything, it's that I didn't tell my children about my cancer until one year later. My youngest, who were 6 and a year old, had no idea that it was cancer, really, but they knew that mommy was sick. But my oldest, who was 11? I should have told him from day one. I didn't, however, because I didn't want him to worry. It was a mistake, though. Why do I regret it? Because he had suspected it all along. He was only 11 years old, but old enough to put two and two together. When he saw me with a bald head, he googled it, talked to his classmates, and *voila*, figured out that his mom had cancer. I still feel quite horrible that he held that knowledge and kept it to himself for an entire year! In other words, he silently suffered and had questions all that time. Kids are extremely smart. Be prepared to talk to them at the onset, in ways that are appropriate for their ages. They'll have a lot of questions and there are tons of great books out there that can help you prepare. One of my favorites was *Because...Someone I love Has Cancer: Kids' Activity Book,* by the American Cancer Society. Your child's pediatrician is a terrific resource as well.
8. A few days after I had received my diagnosis, I was at home lying on the sofa thinking about it all. I was still in disbelief and I didn't know what to do. I'd been to the doctor. I had my results, but I was almost in a state of shock. One of my cousins texted me to ask how I was. We chatted a bit and then she gave me some powerful advice: Just keep moving. That very simple sentence was everything I needed! Just. Keep. Moving. That became my mantra for anytime I felt myself getting stuck or panicky. And so, I pass it along to you. No matter what happens, just keep moving.

CHAPTER 5

The Great Stuart Scott

Before I had breast cancer, I don't think I had any idea who Stuart Scott was. He may have run across my television screen at one point or another, being a well-known ESPN sports broadcaster, but I can't say. But I do know Mr. Scott now and he has become one of my all-time heroes.

In the summer of 2014, Mr. Scott received the Jimmy Valvano award for his perseverance and fight against cancer at the ESPY awards. I stumbled across his speech a few days later and was blown away. It was one of the most courageous, brilliant and inspiring talks that I have ever heard in my life. I carry with me to this day a few things from his speech:

1. "Don't ever give up."
2. "So, live. Live. Fight like hell. And when you get too tired to fight then lay down and rest and let somebody else fight for you."
3. **"When you die, it does not mean that you lose to cancer. You beat cancer by how you live, why you live, and in the manner in which you live."**

That last piece of advice in particular changed my breast cancer life and has become one of my mottoes today. My entire mindset shifted! My entire being! I no longer worried if I was being strong enough or fighting hard enough. I no longer worried if I would just have a miserable existence from here on out. Because, thanks to Mr. Scott, I realized that I could and would take advantage of being yet alive, no matter what! Even if cancer took me out, even if that was my God's will, I would win—meaning cancer wouldn't quite frankly claim my soul, nor my spirit or essence. I would win because I would not merely give up on enjoying whatever I could. I would not just give up. I wouldn't stop *living* while I was yet still *alive.*

Thanks to this new way of thinking I now get so frustrated and even angry whenever I read or hear the standard, go-to phrase "losing their battle with cancer." Are you aware of it? Have you ever been reading a newspaper article or watching television when the reporter so painfully announces that Mrs. X has lost her battle with breast cancer? Have you yourself used it? Maybe I would've used this language, too, if I hadn't heard Mr. Scott's speech.

I *have* heard it, though, and I now realize that we don't have to maintain that defeatist mindset. We don't lose. We don't ever lose because we fight as best we can to maintain our lives *while* we can.

Mr. Scott died not six months after he delivered his speech. I almost can't put into words what it has meant to me. His extremely poignant words gave me the courage and motivation I needed to go forward with cancer and for that, I will forever be grateful to him. I hope with all my heart that he was aware of the light and hope he gave to so many in that speech, especially me.

Chapter 6

Not Everyone Can Take This Journey with You

One of the earliest lessons I learned from having breast cancer is this: Not everyone you know will be able to make this journey with you. Let me repeat that. Not everyone you know will be able make this journey with you. Am I talking about friends? Yes. Coworkers? Yes. Family? Oh, yes. Things could go either way with every single person you know. This is why it is very important to just keep going, with or without the aid of these people.

Once people in my circle—and I have friends and family spread out over the world, from France to Hong Kong—found out that I had breast cancer and that it was serious, reactions varied. My former coworkers at the IT company I worked for at La Défense in Paris rallied around me in ways that I never could have imagined possible. They sent me a signed journal filled with well wishes, raised money for me, and sent flowers. I was and will always be overwhelmed with gratitude. And to think, I had already left the company prior to my diagnosis, and yet they supported me and encouraged me from France.

I received cards, letters, calls, gifts, donations and visits from friends everywhere. I even received donations and gifts from people I barely know. I have been blessed in that I was carried and encouraged and made stronger by these wonderful friends.

Unfortunately, there are a few friends who did not step up as much as I would have liked or thought they would, and you'll experience that, too. That's just life. But remember, you are not alone. I had friends and family whom I had grown up with—whom I'd known for years and years. In the beginning, it hurt me and bothered me to no end, until I decided to stop and refocus. *Never mind, I am not the only one going through this. I have my family. And, there are other breast cancer survivors out there. I am not alone.*

Some of my friends and family members have yet to contact me or call me. Do they care? I don't know. Do they realize how serious it was? I don't know. Will I ask them whenever I see them? No, because at the end of the day you cannot focus on those who are not encouraging you. This will only cause you pain and bring you down. Do. Not. Dwell. On. Anyone. Who. Is. Not. In. Your. Corner. Do not! Pray for them and continue your journey with God's help. Your energy is more important. Keep those who are close to you close, and yes, pray for the ones who are not. We don't know the future. Perhaps God removed them from your journey for a reason. Perhaps he will bring you back together at a later date. Trust in Him.

Sometimes it's not that people aren't in your corner. Sometimes it is as simple as them not knowing what to say or do. When someone is diagnosed with cancer, some people will freeze and worry about saying the wrong thing. So, they say nothing. Please take my advice: If someone in your circle is diagnosed with cancer, say something, even if it is this: "I am sorry you are ill." Or, just simply tell them: "I don't know what to say."

Another thing that can cause you pain and disappointment is to compare yourself to others or compare what one person does for you versus another person. I used to do this all the time until I realized that it is a waste of energy. The problem is this: I know myself and how I would react if someone close to me had cancer. I know that I would try to do whatever is in my power to help them. Visit? You bet. Go to chemotherapy and radiation with them? Absolutely. Take care of their kids? Bring them meals? Clean their house? Hold their hand? Go wig shopping with them? Yes, yes, yes, yes, and yes! Because this is who I am. And because this is who I am, I automatically expected the same from others.

The great news is that I received all of this and more from many, many people. People whom I had just met exceeded my expectations! For example, Natalie, who I met on my new job right when I was diagnosed, took it upon herself to go to our manager and volunteer to take notes for me while I was undergoing chemotherapy, so that I would not get behind in our training. Can you imagine? She had just known me for two weeks. She also gathered cancer information for me, both local and national, with the help of her mother-in-law. She planned a party for me, bought me lots of pink goodies, encouraged me, and called me her hero. In short, she, along with the other people in our group, was a life saver.

Contrast that to a family member whom I considered to be one of my best friends in the entire world. We made plans to talk to each other on the phone, but I could never reach her. I'd leave messages, but she'd never call me back. I was bummed. I felt like I needed her. I wanted her to go with me to chemotherapy or radiation therapy, or help out with my surgery. However, she just wasn't available.

I could not understand why she couldn't be there for me and my family. Did she not understand the gravity of what I was facing? She knew we were newly back to America. She knew we were fighting cancer with half of a job and three children. I am still scratching my head. And because cancer does things to you, changes you in some way, making everything around you more urgent, I was unable to move past her behavior. I stopped trying to call her. I was angry. I was annoyed. But more than anything, I was hurt.

I was devastated.

I tried to come up with excuses for her, but nothing I could think of excused her behavior in my mind. So, I did the only thing I could at the time: I let go. I could not fight that battle along with my breast cancer battle. I could not use the energy on any person who I felt was not in my corner or helping me or my situation. It pained me to do so, but I had to in order to get through it.

I have since spoken to my dear relative (yes, she is still and will forever be dear to me), and I know she still loves me and always has. Even though we have not yet gotten back to where we used to be, I have faith that we will. Open communication and honesty will be key. Sometimes relationships are just out of sync with time and circumstances. Having a potential life-threatening disease is a difficult thing for many people to handle, even if they have the best intentions.

I do not hold grudges and I still have faith that I will be able to rekindle some of the relationships that have suffered since I was diagnosed with cancer. I've also had a lot of time to think about this. I've come to the conclusion that I must forgive whatever perceived slights I encountered. And perceived is a good word here. Maybe I was at fault, too. Maybe I expected too much. No matter what, one thing is certain: no one can quite accurately predict how we will respond to cancer, whether it's ourselves or our loved ones.

Practical Advice for Relationships During Cancer

1. Avoid stress as much as possible.
2. Your number one priority during your cancer journey is focusing on your health—mind, body and spirit. Your healing is all that matters right now. Remember that!
3. Anything or anyone who threatens that needs to be dealt with at a later time. Put non-responsive, toxic or stress-inducing friends and family members on a shelf, at least for now, until you are better and able to look more closely at your relationship. I don't mean that you have to cut people off and out of your life forever. What I am saying is that if you feel someone is not helping you in your journey, pray for them and let them go, at least temporarily. Because the sometimes hard-to-swallow truth is that again, not everyone can go on this journey with you.
4. Stay as close as you can to the people who inspire and encourage you through visits, calls, letters, pep talks, and good deeds. These are your cheerleaders and you need them now more than ever.
5. You will be amazed by the kindness and thoughtfulness of the people with whom you choose to share your journey with. Embrace it, if it helps you.
6. And on the contrary, if you need to take time and space away from people during this journey, do it. People will understand more than you know.

Chapter 7

Cancer Won't Be the Only Thing You're Going Through

It would be easier if this horrific journey were the only thing you had to go through, but unfortunately, it probably won't be. I've met fellow survivors who were going through divorces, custody battles, and abuse. I've met survivors whose children were harming themselves. Another survivor suffered from a mental illness. I've talked to survivors who had just lost their jobs. One woman lost both her parents during the struggle. Some lose their jobs and subsequently their income and can't make ends meet. As you can imagine, the list goes on.

I had my own challenges. For one, my son was still in France with his father and the separation from him was almost unbearable. In addition, my husband couldn't work in the United States because he hadn't received his permanent residence card. Even though I had a job, I couldn't work full-time. Thus, we had about half an income for our entire family. Meanwhile, bills kept rolling in. I thank God that I had just acquired good health insurance, but still, it didn't cover everything. There were co-pays and bills left over. Food, rent, you name it. It was a really tough time for us financially.

On top of all of that was the absolute shock of being back in America as a Black woman after living abroad for almost 16 years. I didn't recognize my country. It was like reverse culture shock when I landed in Maryland. I was utterly lost.

The first time I drove to Johns Hopkins Hospital in downtown Baltimore, this city took my breath away. Not only because I was having my first medical appointment in relation to cancer, but because I was driving by miles and miles of impoverished row houses. It was like being on the set of "The Wire." The scene was shocking.

And then came the death of Michael Brown, followed by Eric Garner, Tamir Rice, Sandra Bland, Walter Scott, Freddie Gray, Philando Castille, and Alton Sterling. These deaths happened during chemotherapy, radiation, surgeries, reconstruction, and physical therapy. These deaths changed the way I thought of America—changed my perception. For you see, while living in Europe, I thought that America had become this place where people of color were more accepted and celebrated. I thought America had evolved. I was horribly wrong, and it saddened me to no end.

I longed to go back to France, but I couldn't because I was in the midst of my treatment. Yet, I was in anguish and pain over what was happening in America. All I could think of was the warning I had received from one of my Franco-American friends in Paris: don't ever go back. He gave me that advice in 2012 when Trayvon Martin was killed. I hadn't listened but, once back, I wish that I had. Things got so bad that I became so anxious, so upset, and so worried that I couldn't sleep at night. I couldn't even drive sometimes for being afraid that I would be pulled over and arrested or worse—shot and killed for no reason. I even hoped that my head scarf or bald head and eyebrow-less face would save me should I be stopped by police. I had a little speech all worked out: "I have breast cancer, Officer. Please don't shoot me."

At that point I knew that I had to do something about these fears, so I stopped watching TV and restricted my social media to updates to friends and family. I simply disconnected myself from the news. Not because I didn't want to know what was happening, but because it was impeding my healing. I could not fight cancer and deal with the systemic racism I saw all around the country at the same time.

I still had to deal with it in person, though. I couldn't escape that.

One day when I arrived for a chemotherapy treatment at Johns Hopkins, I walked into the building's lobby and headed to the elevators.

Standing there waiting was an attractive blond woman who was probably in her fifties. We both got onto the elevator at the same time. What struck me is that as soon as we got on, she huddled herself into one of the corners, then placed her handbag underneath her arm and held it tightly.

My eyes widened. I was saddened by this micro aggression. I was angry. This had not happened to me in all the time I'd lived in France. I couldn't let it slide and so I started a conversation with her.

"I love your bag," I said, looking at her directly.

She smiled and seemed to clutch it tighter.

"Did you buy it in Paris or in the United States?" I continued.

"I bought it in Paris," she answered, seemingly surprised at the question.

"Did you get it at the flagship store on the Champs-Élysées?" I asked.

Her jaw dropped. "I sure did!" she said with a smile.

"Yes, most of the tourists shop there," I said, smiling back as politely as I could, although I was seething because not a minute earlier this woman was convinced that I might try to snatch her Louis Vuitton.

"How did you know?" she asked. "Have you been to that store?"

"Yes, many times. I just moved back from Paris," I said.

She loosened her grip on the bag and dropped it down to her side.

I was boiling inside.

"That must have been quite an experience…" Blah blah blah.

I didn't hear a word she said afterwards. I just stood there waiting for the elevator doors to open so I could escape. I didn't care what floor it was stopping on. I just knew I wanted to get as far away from that woman as possible.

When I finally got to my floor I smiled and said something like, "Have a nice day," then made my way to the chemotherapy bay.

She waved and as sweetly as a new best friend, saying, "You too, honey. You take care now."

I was still livid, but I knew I had to shake it off. I had to put it in a box with the utterly heartbreaking images that I'd seen on television of Eric

Garner begging for his life. I had to get myself together for another face off with the Red Devil, also known as Adriamycin. This chemotherapy drug is a formidable foe. I had to be ready mentally, emotionally and spiritually. That's all that mattered.

And this is all that should matter when you are going through your cancer journey: block out everything that impedes your healing and progress. As I write this today, thousands of people from not only the United States, but around the world in large cities such as Paris, Toronto, London and Berlin are marching in the streets. They are marching because there has been another killing, the murder of an African-American man named George Floyd, who died on video screaming for his momma as a white Minnesota policeman kept his knee on his neck (while three other officers held him down) until he breathed his last breath. The outrage of his murder has spread around the entire world.

Yet, as tired as I am, as gutted as I am, I have no choice but to take the same advice that I am about to give you. Whether it's your own crisis, distraction, racism, culture shock, divorce, job loss, family and or financial issues—set it aside. What you are enduring right now, especially if you are in the thick of your treatment, will require your very best efforts. Be mindful of any negative energy and keep positive energy around you as much as you can. I am convinced that a positive mindset played a vital role in my healing. It will in yours as well.

Practical Advice for Focusing on Your Health

1. It's all about YOU! You might not be used to putting yourself first, but during cancer, you absolutely must. So, repeat after me: **"It's all about me!"**
2. Set aside anything or anyone that is causing you stress, strife or emotional (and physical) harm. You must focus on yourself right now.
3. Know that your mental, spiritual and emotional well-being are just as important as your physical well-being.
4. Cancer discombobulates you, your family, and your life. Guard against your mental health.
5. That being said, point out at least one positive thing in your life every single day. Jot it down on a small piece of paper and put it in an old mason jar, box or other container. Read over these pieces of encouragement whenever things seem dark or you find yourself slipping.
6. Don't get so caught up in world events (racism, politics, storms, floods, etc.) that you cease to function—that you become distracted from your number one priority: getting better!
7. If there are situations that require an important decision, try to postpone it until your treatment is over. I contemplated moving back to Paris, but I knew that going back in the middle of chemotherapy wasn't the right time to make that choice.
8. Getting cancer is not your fault and do not blame yourself for the illness or your needs. I have met other survivors who

ended up in the middle of a divorce due to their illness. In addition, I once talked to a survivor whose family had castigated and left her to her own devices because they thought she was too "needy."

9. Again, if something is impeding your healing, put it aside until you can handle it. For me, I had to turn off the news and stop scrolling on Twitter, lest I see the videos of Eric Garner (and others) again. I knew that I could not handle that heartbreak anymore.
10. If you have financial difficulties, talk to your bank and lenders. Many of them will work with you if they know what your situation is. Keeping them in the loop is key. Another possibility is GoFundMe, which allows people to contribute money to you, whether they're strangers or family. Many of your friends and family will especially appreciate this because it provides them with a very easy way to help you.
11. In addition, talk to social workers and the financial manager at the hospital. In one instance I received assistance for my Neulasta shot, which at the time cost $8200 per shot.
12. And don't forget to talk to the nurses in the chemotherapy bay. My nurses at Johns Hopkins were an excellent source and shared a lot of information with me that I would not have known about otherwise. Some of the things I benefitted from thanks to various organizations and associations were gas cards, grocery cards, free maid service, cash gifts, free head scarfs and blankets, and more.
13. Don't be afraid to find other organizations and associations and ask them for help. If you cannot perform the research, ask someone to do it for you. As I mentioned, a good friend took it upon herself and did this for me. She came back with a

pretty extensive local and national list, which ended up being incredibly helpful.

14. And again, because I cannot say this enough: NEVER BLAME YOURSELF. Cancer is not your fault.
15. Breathe and take one day at a time.
16. Go back and read number one again.

CHAPTER 8

Surviving Chemotherapy

Chemo: who hasn't heard the horror stories? If you want to give someone the shivers, just mention the word. I had no idea how I was going to get through it, just that I had to get through it.

I remember quite vividly my sessions, especially the earlier ones. After the first round of ACT (Adriamycin, Cytoxan and Taxol) had gone rather well, considering, I arrived at my second one feeling optimistic, but still fearful that it would go downhill at any moment.

I signed in, took a seat, and saw Dr. F. Strangely enough I felt excited, maybe because I was doing this thing. I stared at him and smiled because he reminded me of my college mentor, Dr. Tatham. Dr. F. sat in front of me and asked how I was doing. I was encouraged and ready to battle. I got my vitals taken and found out that I had gained weight. Yowzah! I knew my pants were tighter. I made a mental note: work out! And then a second one: lay off the fried foods! Since I'd been back in the U.S., Taco Bell, Burger King and Chick-fil-A were consistently calling my name. My third mental note was this: note #2 does not apply during ACT because with my first cycle of chemo, I craved chicken and Chipotle and all things spicy. I looked forward to getting through that treatment and getting my hands on something piquant!

The doctor had discussed the side effects. He said I might not suffer from all of them, but in addition to food cravings, I certainly suffered from others—including fatigue, nausea, headaches, sore mouth, itchiness, flu-like symptoms and achiness. Besides dealing with overall fear and the effects of the powerful drugs in my chemo regimen, I was concerned about losing my hair.

I'd been natural for a couple of years and had finally grown my hair into an awesome Afro. That was about to change, according to the doctors. Chemotherapy would make every single hair on my head fall out. That saddened me, but I was determined not to let it break me.

My first chemo treatment took place on July 8, and 19 days later my hair started falling out. Even my eyelashes were falling and sticking to my lenses. Like much that I would experience during this journey, it was surreal. My hair continued to fall out little by little for an entire week. If I ran my hand through it, it would fall into the sink. I started seeing spots and wider spaces. "Argh," was my response. It was impressive and destabilizing all at once. I didn't know how many more days until I was completely bald. I wasn't ready.

But I had to be.

I decided to take control of the situation and not wait for my hair to fall into my hands in huge chunks. (I'd read too many terrible stories about that and did not want to put myself in that situation.) I came home from work that day and asked my husband to shave it. I ended up with a super short hairdo, less than half an inch, but I was relieved. Having my beautiful locks running into the shower drain was not going to be one of the nightmares I had.

It was a great decision except my four-year-old wasn't ready for it either. I failed to explain what Mommy and Daddy were doing, and why, so she freaked out. If you decide to shave your hair, make sure you explain it to your children beforehand so that you don't shock them.

The morning after I felt that I still maintained some sense of control over my life, and my looks. I still had a say. I could still have a *when*. And besides, the super short hairdo looked quite good on me.

Of course, it didn't take long for even that hair to start falling out, and even though it was super short, the effect was shocking. Even though you know what to expect, it is still unnerving and disaffecting. By this time, I had already amassed 30 or so scarves. I was determined to look my best, still, on my new job. Oh, did I mention I was still working? I was trying my best to live as much of a normal life as I could, even though my body was under full attack from the cancer and the toxins being pumped into my body to get rid of it.

Not only did I lose my hair, but all of my nails turned a dark blue-black color. My taste buds died, and I suffered from an extremely dry mouth. I had hot flashes during the day and night, which made me miserable. To top it all off, I experienced the onset of medical menopause. Now, I wasn't upset about that. I already had three children. However, the fact that the drugs were strong enough to cause that made me freak out all the same.

Even with all the effects taking place in my mind and body, the chemotherapy itself was fairly tolerable for me. If you didn't know me, aside from the bald head that I kept covered up, you wouldn't ever guess that I was undergoing treatment. I didn't lose weight. I was able to eat most of the time. I was able to walk without trouble most days and I even played tennis a couple of times. And, I was able to work, although sometimes it was a challenge. From a mental standpoint, I remained positive and happy and upbeat whenever I went into the chemo bay as best I could. Let me repeat that: as best I could.

But I sat next to people who were not doing so well. Who were not upbeat, who were not positive, who were not tolerating the drugs very well. I sat next to people who looked sick.

I never looked sick during my cancer treatment.

Which brings me to this: please be aware that cancer does not look the same on everyone. I repeat, cancer does not look the same on everyone. That means, your journey will be different. Your body will be different. How you look and feel might be different. Every single cancer case is different. People can share their experiences with you, but it doesn't mean that you will have the exact same journey.

I learned a lot through chemotherapy. It was an eye opener for me in many ways. Not only did I learn a lot about myself, I also learned a lot about cancer, and suffering, and the human spirit.

My personal mantra was that I wanted to maintain a positive mindset during all of my treatment, especially chemotherapy, because I thought it would be the hardest part of my treatment.

However, not everyone can do that.

There is such a thing as chemotherapy etiquette. Yes! Indeed, there is. If you should find yourself accompanying someone during their treatment or if you yourself have to undergo treatment, here are a few things to keep in mind, things that I learned along the way.

Practical Advice for Chemotherapy

1. Take a family member or a friend with you to treatments, if possible. But make sure they know they're going for something that will be difficult. Not everyone can stomach the chemotherapy bay.
2. If you have to go alone or prefer to, take a book, your iPad or laptop to pass the time. You're going to be there for a few hours. TVs are available in some places—there was one in mine. Sometimes you might find yourself too nauseous to watch it, though.
3. If you are able to eat, take something with you. You don't want to become weaker from lack of food during the treatment. There might be snacks available for you in the chemo bay, too.
4. Regarding other patients, don't stare at other people sitting in the chemotherapy bay with you. Some people are extremely guarded and discreet and do not want that.
5. Be nice to your nursing staff. They have tough jobs and a kind word with them goes a very long way.
6. Don't ask people what type of cancer they have, or what round of chemo they're on.
7. Please don't take in smelly food. That Chinese food, chicken curry, even popcorn will certainly make most patients nauseous.
8. Don't talk/laugh loudly. Sorry, but people don't want to hear about your beach vacation, son's breakup (no matter how juicy the details) or your colonoscopy!
9. Chemotherapy is a delicate thing. Most people are tired, achy, sickly and just don't want to be there. The last thing you want to

do is answer a lot of questions or overhear loud conversations. You want the atmosphere to be as peaceful as it can be.

10. If you have any doubts about what to do, err on the side of caution. Refrain from probing questions; don't force conversation.
11. Regarding hair loss: yes, as I have stated, you will lose it, but remember, you are defined by other things, too. Your hair will grow back. Now you get to experiment with wigs. Ever wanted to go blonde? Love red hair? Long hair? Short hair? The sky's the limit! Also, some insurances will pay for one wig during your treatment. Inquire.
12. Be careful eating a lot of what you love (if you can eat) during chemotherapy. I ate tons of frozen yogurt because one, I love it, and two, it was one of the few things I actually could eat. But to this day, eating frozen yogurt remains difficult. Why? It's an automatic association with the treatment. Someone had warned me about it, but unfortunately it was too late.
13. If you have a port-a-cath, or a "port," your healthcare team can easily access your vein in order to receive your chemo. The great thing about this is that you won't endure countless needle sticks each time. I do recommend that you get one if your doctor agrees in order to receive your chemo. Also, don't forget to get an EMLA cream prescription before your first session and apply it an hour or so before your treatment. This numbing cream is awesome. By applying it, you won't feel any "sticks." I forgot it one time, learned my lesson, and never forgot it again.
14. "Chemo brain" is real. I know this for a fact, and I've discussed it with my doctor. There's a sort of brain fog that you get during or after your treatment. Mine started sometime after my treatments had ended. I found out I had it like this: One day my husband recounted something that I had no memory of telling him, not one. But I knew that he couldn't have known it without

me giving him the information. Try as I might, I had absolutely no recollection of the conversation. Was it scary? Absolutely! And this happened more than a few times.

15. How intense or how long "chemo brain" will last depends on each person. In the meantime, take notes. Write everything down. Take brain quizzes and do mental exercises. It does get better.
16. Chemotherapy is definitely a challenge and I don't ever want to go through it again. It is tough, but you can do this. Just take one treatment at a time. I repeat, take one treatment at a time.

Chapter 9

Losing a Part of Me: The Mastectomy

After all the tests—biopsies, MRIs, PET-CT scans—my breast surgeon concluded that I needed a mastectomy. I guess I had rather expected it and when he told me, I said, "If it will save my life, cut it off." First, I underwent neoadjuvant treatment—I had all of my chemotherapy before surgery. This treatment consisted of five months of intensive chemotherapy and half of my target therapy sessions. Therefore, I had time to think about the mastectomy.

Now, don't get me wrong. It wasn't like I was in a hurry to have a part of me surgically removed. I wasn't. It was so unreal, like my entire cancer experience. I decided to write about it, because that's what I do: I write, and it helps me get my feelings out. So, I wrote this piece, which was published in The Washington Post, entitled, "Already Missing a Part of Me on the Eve of My Mastectomy." That piece summed up what I was feeling right before my surgery: reflective, scared, anxious, and appreciative of what I'd had in terms of my body *before* cancer.

On the eve of my mastectomy, I just couldn't believe it. I couldn't believe that I had endured months of chemotherapy and was now having a mastectomy to remove one of my breasts. I was put to sleep, operated on, and when I woke up, that breast was gone forever. It's not that I wanted to do it, but the cancer had made it impossible to continue living with that part of my body. I wish it could have been different. Why did I cancel all those appointments for mammograms? Why, oh why, oh why? It was too late to ask that question and it doesn't help to ask it today, either. But the fact does remain that if I had caught this disease earlier, maybe just a small part of my breast would have been removed.

Breasts are breasts. They're just an ordinary body part, right? Yes. And then no, not really. Some women love theirs; others hate theirs. Some just don't care. I had always been so happy with mine. I never considered them to be too small, or too large. Before pregnancies, during pregnancies, and after the birth of each of my three children, I could always count on my breasts to bounce back and be the perfect pair that they were.

I had never allowed others to call them silly names like "ta-tas." I had always given them firm support throughout our life together. When I moved to Paris, I was in heaven when I shopped in luxurious lingerie stores such as Aubade and La Perla. Nothing was too good for them, but now, I would only have one.

I wasn't so worried about the operation, but I was worried about how I would feel after I woke up and my breast was gone.

It's weird, still, that it's gone. Since the surgery, I have had reconstruction and although I have come a long way, my breast still isn't the same and I now know that it never will be. I guess I am okay with that. I guess I have to be. I don't know if I truly appreciated having two "normal" breasts as much as I do now.

It's a strange thing to walk around wondering whether or not people can look at you and spot that one of your breasts is different from the other one—that one is bigger or less round. In the beginning, I was self-conscious sometimes. At other times, I didn't care.

I like to remind myself time and time again—at least I am still here. That's one of my other new life mottos, in case you haven't noticed. At least I am *still here.* And if you are reading this, *you* are still here. Whether you have one breast now or two, you are still a woman. You are still a female. You are mothers, wives, sisters, daughters, and best friends. Having one less breast (or none!) doesn't have to change who we are.

Strive to live your life to the fullest—to dance, sing, run, play, go to the beach—to do all of the things you've been doing up until now, no matter what.

Practical Advice for a Mastectomy

1. Don't forget to take an extra-large shirt that buttons in the front and a pair of comfy elastic-waist pants for when you leave the hospital. The bigger the shirt the better, as you likely will be leaving with drainage tubes ("drains"). Some people opt for special shirts with drain pockets or pouches. I pinned them to my pants and, with my big shirt pulled down over them, no one was the wiser.
2. You will definitely need assistance after your surgery, so try to arrange for a friend or loved one to help you once you get home.
3. If you don't have anyone available to assist you, prepare as best you can before entering into the hospital for the surgery. For example: shop for and prepare food that will be easy to reheat; place household objects at eye level so you won't have to stretch your arm.
4. Once you get back home, rest. You will need lots of it. Don't try to do too much too soon.
5. Don't be afraid to ask for help when it comes to childcare, cleaning, laundry, and shopping.
6. Be careful not to get your drains hung up on things within your house. I once got one of my drain tubes stuck on a doorknob. Trust me, that really hurt. I pinned my drains to my pants in order to prevent that from happening again.
7. Take your meds! Always stay on top of those and don't wait until the pain catches up with you.

8. Some women will want to keep their mastectomies private, and that's okay, too.
9. Be kind and gentle to yourself. You've just endured something very challenging and difficult. Allow yourself time to heal.

Chapter 10

Reconstruction and My New Breast

Before the mastectomy, I met with my breast surgeon to discuss reconstructive options. The implant appealed to me most. Although I didn't get any advice from other women who had breast cancer, I spoke to a few who had breast implants to glean more information. During my mastectomy, the surgeon put in a tissue expander—a temporary breast implant filled with saline solution that expanded my breast tissue and muscle and kept them stretched out until I could get a regular breast implant. Sometimes these are painful, but I am fortunate that my implant didn't cause me any trouble. After healing, it was time for the next step: reconstruction.

When looking at a more permanent solution, I thought I'd go with a breast implant, but then I learned about the DIEP flap surgery (deep inferior epigastric perforator flap) and thought that might be a good idea, also. However, the amount of recovery time scared me: 6-8 weeks. I met with a reconstructive surgeon who informed me that due to the radiation I'd had, it would not be possible nor advisable for me to have an implant. He recommended a DIEP flap surgeon and that was that.

Even though I was still nervous about the recovery time, I was somewhat happy that I wouldn't have a foreign implant in my body for the rest of my life. The expander, I was afraid, would burst or get infected. But remember, every choice in your breast cancer journey is yours and yours alone; it's extremely personal. What worked for me might not work for you, and that's perfectly normal and okay.

The DIEP flap surgery is an advanced microsurgical technique that is used to rebuild your breast. It is a serious surgery that will challenge you mentally, physically and emotionally. During my reconstructive surgery, the doctor took excess living fat from below the belly button (my tummy) and transplanted it to my chest to create a new breast. One of the main things fellow survivors ask me when it comes to reconstruction is: "Was it worth it and would you do it again?" The answer is overwhelmingly, "YES!"

I was fortunate to have an excellent doctor (with an excellent bedside manner, to boot). I was operated on three times: once for the initial DIEP flap, and then twice afterwards to have additional fat transfers to help with the size and shape of the breast. Every surgery was a success, thankfully.

The initial surgery was the hardest. After the operation, I was in the ICU unit for a couple of days (standard procedure). My entire hospital stay probably lasted about five days. After the procedure, I could not get out of bed by myself. I could not get up and go to the bathroom and had to be accompanied by a nurse. It took a few days for me to be able to walk again. After starting on a walker, each day got easier and easier. But I was flabbergasted at how immobile I had become. From one day to the next, I was yet again a different person, having to rely on someone else just to get out of bed.

I healed, though, and so will you. It's a huge operation, but I feel like it was so worth it.

At some time during your recovery or afterwards, someone will eventually make the comment that "at least you got a free tummy tuck" during your reconstructive surgery. They'll see your flatter belly and envy you. That's because when you have this surgery, it's sort of like getting a "tummy tuck" because your body will also benefit from an improved abdominal shape. The reason is the doctor uses fat from your belly to create the new breast, thereby giving you a tighter abdomen. You'll probably look at the person and think they're insane, of course, because who wants a "tummy tuck" under these circumstances? Who wants a "tummy tuck" due to cancer, mastectomy and a reconstruction? Right, no one. At this point, you'll just have to ignore them (or not) and hope they one day realize that we would have much rather kept our original breasts to begin with!

This surgery left me with a dark scar that runs from hip to hip, and it still itches like crazy sometimes, but that's acceptable to me. My doctor was able to recreate a part of me that I thought I had lost forever. It's not exactly like it was before cancer and the mastectomy, but it's better than I could have ever expected.

Practical Advice for Reconstructive Surgery

1. If you decide to have the DIEP flap surgery, make sure you find a doctor who specializes in this type of procedure.
2. As with the mastectomy, you'll definitely need assistance after your hospital stay. The reconstructive surgery was more challenging (physically) than my mastectomy. Everyone is different, of course, so pay attention to your body and your own needs.
3. As with the mastectomy, don't forget to take an extra-large shirt that buttons in the front and a pair of comfy elastic-waist pants with you for when you leave the hospital. Yes, you'll have drains again—sorry, but they come with the territory. With this surgery, I kept them longer than I did with the mastectomy, as it took longer for all the fluids to filter out.
4. Having a pillow in your car will certainly help when you leave the hospital.
5. You won't be able to drive for two to three weeks. I was able to go back to work in five weeks. Expect that it will take you between four and six weeks to fully recover.
6. You will need additional surgeries with more fat transfers after the initial surgery in order to get the size/shape you want. I stopped after two fat transfers (third overall surgery) because I moved to a new state and didn't want to start over with another doctor. I feel that I need a couple of more fat transfers, but I just don't feel up to it. Maybe one day, I'll continue—or this size will be it.

7. One of the most important tips that I can give you is don't let yourself get constipated. Painkillers will do that to you. Make sure you don't let this get out of hand. I was so miserable. For me, this was worse than any pain that I had with the surgeries. I'm sure it's not an especially great memory for my husband who had the unlucky task of giving me an enema, which is why I'll probably never leave him (insert LOL here).
8. Don't be surprised if someone tells you that you are lucky to have gotten a tummy tuck out of your breast cancer and reconstructive experience. Kindly explain that you would have preferred to have a tummy tuck WITHOUT THE CANCER.

CHAPTER 11

The Fog of Radiation Therapy

By the time I'd had radiation, I'd already undergone months of chemotherapy, targeted therapy and my mastectomy. I felt like I was on the other side of the hill, beginning the descent when it comes to treatment.

Much of what I went through is somewhat as foggy today as it was then, but what I can tell you is that compared to chemotherapy, radiation felt so much easier. Now, don't get me wrong; radiation therapy is a very serious thing in itself. But at the time it felt more manageable to me than the chemo drugs. Was it in the end? I'm unsure.

I had some side effects that lasted a long time after my 35 sessions or so had finished. For example, I developed Lymphedema (although I don't know if it was a direct result of radiation therapy or the removal of some lymph nodes), and my skin in the breast area and shoulder turned black. It eventually returned to its normal color, but it took a while; my shoulder, arm and breast area remain to this day very tight and I need to stretch them out often. Fatigue was another side effect.

But at the time of my treatment, which was eight months after I had been diagnosed, I was so much more at ease. I was still having the targeted therapy (Herceptin + Perjeta), but at least chemotherapy was over. I was ecstatic to begin this new phase of healing.

I went to the hospital five days a week for about six weeks. All of the appointments were incredibly short, and I was usually in and out within 20 minutes. The atmosphere was different from that of the chemotherapy bay. It seemed lighter, easier. On the other hand, maybe that was just how I was feeling because I was done with chemo.

Once the radiation team called me back to the radiation room, I had to lie down and position my arm in a slightly uncomfortable position; I managed. I had to lie incredibly still because the radiation therapy machine was aiming specific amounts of radiation at my breast area in order to kill cancer cells or keep them from spreading.

My choice of music, which was usually Bach or Beethoven, played in the background and aided in getting me through all of these sessions.

The time flew by and before I knew it, I was I ringing the bell at the end, in the same way that I had done in chemotherapy. I was so grateful that another phase was over.

Practical Advice for Radiation Therapy

1. You'll have a ton of questions to ask your doctor about this new phase of your treatment. Don't be shy. The main questions that I wanted to know were when, why (although my oncologist had explained it), how and for how long.
2. Ask about all the risks and side effects—both long term and short term. My doctor gave me a list and I consult it from time to time even now.
3. They'll certainly tell you how to prepare for radiation and alert you to what you can and cannot do during your treatment.
4. Wearing loose-fitting clothes to each session is a good idea, especially when it comes to the top half of your body.
5. Keep the area clean with fragrance-free soaps that contain moisturizer. I used Dove.
6. Do not take hot showers during this time (that was hard, but I got used to it).
7. Do not use a razor on that side of the body.
8. A moisturizer will become one of your new best friends. Make sure you moisturize after every treatment and long afterwards. I recommend Aquaphor or Eucerin.
9. Along those lines, ask your doctor about the usage of sunscreen. However, the best thing to do especially during treatment is to keep the affected area covered up (your entire shoulder and part of your back and neck). I also use plenty of sunscreen whenever I go to the beach now.

10. Be mindful of fatigue. I tried to maintain work during the entire course of treatment, but near the end, the fatigue just caught up to me. It can come out of nowhere. Pace yourself and get as much rest as you can. Even though you may feel that you're perfectly fine, your body is undergoing a very serious treatment.

CHAPTER 12:

If You Develop Lymphedema...

After surviving all of my treatment and the cancer itself, I developed lymphedema. CancerCenters.com defines lymphedema as: "swelling caused by the excess buildup of fluid under the skin and is often caused when lymph nodes are removed or damaged. The lymph nodes act as a filter for waste, which is swept up and carried to the lymph nodes by the protein-rich lymphatic fluid. When the lymph nodes are damaged or blocked, the lymphatic fluid may accumulate beneath the skin in the lymph vessels and cause gradual swelling."

There are two types of this condition:

- Primary lymphedema, which is rare, is a genetic condition in which the lymph nodes or vessels are missing or aren't fully developed.
- Secondary lymphedema, which is caused by another condition that damages the lymph nodes or vessels, may be caused by a lymph node infection, cancer, radiation, surgery or injury (which is what I have).

Curiously enough, my lymphedema didn't start immediately. In fact, it didn't start until the summer of 2018, which was four years after I was diagnosed with breast cancer. There I was, thinking that I had escaped that particular fate, but no. I hadn't. One day I arrived at work only to find that one of my hands looked like the Incredible Hulk's. The lymphedema probably resulted from my breast surgeon having to remove 10 of my lymph nodes during surgery. It could also be from radiation therapy, or a combination of the two. In any case, my arm now swells a little, and my hand swells a lot.

Because of that, I have to wear a compression sleeve for the rest of my life to avoid the swelling. After trying many different types of garments,

I was successful in finding one that works well for me. The sleeves can be off the shelf (if you have a mild case) or customized for your specific needs, which is my case.

Unfortunately, lymphedema becomes a part of our journey and it's more noticeable sometimes than the other scars because of the sleeve and glove comb that I wear. I used to have a job in which I interviewed upwards of 40 people daily. Oh, the questions they had about my sleeve/glove. If only I had a dollar for every one. If you're wearing a compression garment every day, expect people to ask if you've been burned, have carpal tunnel syndrome, or have a sports injury. I'd say that one out of 100 correctly guessed why I wear it.

Don't feel compelled to discuss it. In the beginning, I would explain and go through the entire breast cancer story until finally, I got tired of it. I credit this one rude person with waking me up to the fact that hey, I don't have to share everything with everyone. A guy I was interviewing one day tried to guess why I was wearing my sleeve and he guessed incorrectly each time. When I got tired and told him why, he couldn't stop talking about how horrible it must be, how hot, how bothersome, and on and on and on. That day I made a decision to either tell people that it was lymphedema (and educate them a little) or I'd just say, "It's a long story." You decide what's best for you.

I know none of this is optimal. It's hard. You might be angry and bitter about it, and that's okay. I was a little bitter and angry, too, and some days, I'm utterly sad. I have never spoken to other women who've developed lymphedema due to breast cancer, nor have I had any counseling, but I don't doubt that it could be useful. Apparently anger and frustration from being left with this chronic illness after everything else we've been through is very common. It's definitely understandable. Lymphedema sometimes seems like a second punishment after all the treatments, surgeries, and mental anguish. The most important thing you can do is to keep taking care of yourself, get a good sleeve (this is vital), and live life as normally as you possibly can.

The sleeve that I've had success with (after trying several different kinds) is the Medi Mondi Esprit one-piece unit. Because I endure swelling in my hand, the two pieces (sleeve plus a gauntlet) did not work for me. Try different options until you find the right one.

Lymphedema will change your life and exact certain demands, but hasn't everything you've gone through with breast cancer? Chalk it up as another part of your new life post-breast cancer.

At least I'm still here. I use my motto whenever I need to.

Practical Advice Regarding Lymphedema

1. If you develop lymphedema, take extra good care of the infected arm/hand.
2. One of the most important things is finding the sleeve that works for you. Not everyone's swelling is the same. If you need a customized fit, have your therapist or doctor measure you for one.
3. Don't be afraid to experiment until you find that right combination. You might feel some frustration going through this process, but once you find the right sleeve, the rest is just routine maintenance.
4. You might need a nighttime glove—a huge sleeve that looks like an oven mitt! Ask your doctor.
5. Please be mindful that you can't sleep in the daytime sleeve. Ask your doctor for the nighttime sleeve.
6. You CAN wear the nighttime sleeve during the day—if your swelling is controlled.
7. Exercise and lowering your salt intake can help with your swelling.
8. When you wear a compression garment, expect people to ask if you've been burned, have carpal tunnel syndrome, or have a sports injury. Be prepared to answer them or not. It's entirely your decision. Don't feel compelled to discuss it.
9. In the beginning of your diagnosis, make notes about your swelling. For example, I now know that I can go a whole day without my sleeve and not have serious consequences. I know that I can skip my nighttime glove about three nights before

there's a noticeable amount of swelling. So, monitor your situation and work within your limits. Everyone is different.

10. Do not put your compression garments in the dryer (even though some nighttime sleeves are allowed). Better to air dry them all. Always use a garment bag to wash them in as well.
11. If possible, you will need two daytime sleeves because you need to wash your sleeve daily so that the original shape returns (for this reason, I recommend having two sleeves at least). I am currently working with four daytime sleeves just to make it easier.
12. If your insurance allows, get a lymphedema pump. I currently use the Flexi-touch Plus for one hour a day. This machine moves lymph fluid around the body through gentle massage. I used to groan about "going on the pump," as we call it in my house. Now I look forward to this hour every night. I can watch Netflix, read or just relax while managing my lymphedema at the same time. Again, look for the positive things.
13. It is annoying sometimes, but wear your sleeve, moisturize and take good care of your arm/hand, and keep it moving.
14. Join a lymphedema and a breast cancer support group (there are plenty on Facebook) where you can share tips with and seek support from fellow survivors. This is also a wonderful way to collectively share our experiences and help to mitigate the anger. The ability to talk about the problem with people who know exactly what you're going through is an important step toward acceptance.

Chapter 13

Life After Cancer: Your New Normal

Having a "new normal" after breast cancer is something that we all have to come to terms with eventually. When I first heard this expression, I disliked it. It frightened me. I didn't want a new normal. I just wanted normal. I wanted my old life back, my pre-cancer life. It's called new normal because things won't ever be the same for you. But trust me, that's okay—and it's not as scary as it sounds.

I felt like my new normal began the moment I learned that I had breast cancer. First, I was plagued by the thought that I might possibly die, leaving behind my husband and my three young children. That fear can be all-consuming. That fear can cause you to want to jump into bed, put your head under the covers and never come out again.

There are physical ailments and effects that linger from radiation and/or chemo, your surgeries, lymphedema. Is it fair? Absolutely not! Is it *chiante*, as we say in France? Totally! Can these things stop you from living your best life? Maybe, but it depends. Just as everyone's cancer diagnosis is different, so is everyone's new normal.

I've talked about my lymphedema, but my new normal also includes "phantom" itching. Phantom itching means that I can feel something itching just beneath the surface, but I can't seem to get to it to scratch it. I feel this in my reconstructed breast and it's due to the mastectomy. I also have phantom itching where my DIEP scar is. That one's the worst and keeps me up a little from time to time. It has gotten much better over the years.

I also still experience fatigue, chemo brain, and other aches and pains here and there. But the most challenging effect can be found within your own mind, and that is the fear of recurrence.

After I'd completed all my treatments from A to Z, I was left with confronting my fears of recurrence. My doctor does not prescribe routine PET/CT scans or MRIs to check for signs of cancer, but I still meet with him quarterly for a physical checkup and I know to contact him immediately if I develop any worrisome symptoms.

When I look back on how I felt, say, three years ago, versus now, I can see that I've come a long way, and you will also. Every day that you are here decreases the chances of recurrence.

When I let myself really get to a place of doubt, I remember Stuart Scott and his tremendous courage. I also remember that I am already winning. Furthermore, I remind you of this extremely important lesson that I learned early on in this fight against cancer and all that it entails: If you are always worried about dying, then you cannot and will not truly live.

Right now, there is a global pandemic happening and the term "new normal" has been used quite a lot. We must wear masks. We must stay six feet apart from each other (social distancing). We must not meet in crowds...and so on. Well, as a breast cancer survivor, I am already used to having a "new normal," so when I initially heard that, I wanted to say, "Ha! I don't have any problems with a 'new normal!' Take that, coronavirus!" Instead, what I really said was, "OK, I can do this."

And, so can you.

Living in the midst of a pandemic certainly makes our "new normal" more challenging, but we can do this. We are already doing it! So, try not to be too afraid of this term. Don't let it intimidate you.

Instead, live! Live the best life you can while you can. No one asks for cancer. No one knows the future, and no one apart from another survivor will understand exactly what you have been through. But that's okay. You're still here and being here gives you yet another chance to smile, to love, and to share. Every single day is a gift and a chance to begin again. You might not have the best attitude or outlook every day, but that's alright, too. You wouldn't be human if you didn't fall down sometimes. However, you don't have to stay down. Take your life by the horns, whatever that looks like for you right now, and keep it moving. You are the author of your own story, and how you decide to live from this day forward is up to you. No matter what happens, you are brave, you are loved, and you are a survivor. No matter what.

Practical Advice for Living Your New Normal

1. First, you must fully understand that life *after* cancer is different than life *before* cancer. You might not ever get to the same point you were before you were sick, and that's okay. A new normal gives you the opportunity to start over.
2. You've been through a lot. Be patient and give yourself time to recover.
3. Everyone is different and processes it differently, but you'll likely experience different emotions once your treatment ends. Don't worry. This is all normal. You've been practically attached to your medical team for months, and once everything stops or slows down, we are sometimes left a little lost.
4. When it comes to recurrence:
    a. Recurrence anxiety is real but remember this: If you are too busy worrying about dying, you cannot or will not truly *live*.
    b. If you weren't eating healthy or exercising before, now is the time to start. This is not only good in terms of keeping cancer from coming back, but it's good for your overall health.
    c. Try to arrive at and maintain a healthy weight.
    d. Avoid drinking excessive alcohol.
    e. Do I even need to mention smoking? If you do, stop!
    f. Drink lots of water and stay away from excessive amounts of junk food.
    g. Speak to a professional therapist if you find yourself stuck on these thoughts and unable to function. This is important!
5. If you're still experiencing side effects, let your medical team know.

6. Share your experiences with other survivors. You can give back by answering questions and giving your own advice through online forums such as Facebook and other groups. It can really help them and you.
7. Don't be ashamed of your scars: If it makes you feel more comfortable, talk about your experiences with people you care about before they see your scars. Someone who truly cares about you won't care, and for those who dislike your scars, tell them to get lost! You are beautiful regardless. You are a warrior! You are a goddess, my friend.
8. It's okay if you don't have a grand epiphany after your experience or some urgent vows to change your life.
9. Love yourself and congratulate yourself that you've come this far.
10. If people around you die from cancer, you will probably feel a more intense sense of loss. I have lost two friends to cancer since I was diagnosed, one to brain cancer and the other to breast cancer. It is hard. It is *very* hard. Your brain will ask you questions, like, why them? Why not me? How was I spared? Am I next? If you start dwelling on recurrence, go back and read #4. Regardless, you must keep going. You must remember that every cancer case is different. Continue and honor the people you lose.
11. Believe it or not, there are some positive things that can come out of cancer. For me, I felt stronger, and closer to God, family and friends.
12. Keep in mind what Stuart Scott said: You win no matter what, by living your life to the fullest while you can.

CHAPTER 14

How My Personal Faith Saved Me

While you most certainly will need to look within yourself and find strength that you never knew you had (and you can and will!), you can also look beyond yourself. I grew up in a Christian environment. I attended church at least twice a week with my grandparents, including Sunday School and Wednesday-night prayer services. During cancer, I found that I needed God more than ever, and He was there for me. In fact, I know that He was there for me from the beginning. Therefore, I would be remiss not to give my personal testimony here.

It blows my mind when I think about how perfectly orchestrated it all was. Imagine this: my French company was bought out, causing my department to be closed and my entire team fired. Because of that, I searched for and found a new job in America, and my family and I decided to move. As I was packing up, I came across an old doctor's order. I had received it at my six-week checkup after my third child was born. When I found it, it was one month from expiring. Since I didn't know when my new health insurance would kick in, I scheduled an appointment for the mammogram, thinking that I would get it over with before leaving France. And that's how I found out that I had breast cancer.

But it doesn't end there.

My new job was located in Baltimore, Maryland, which is the home of Johns Hopkins Hospital, which happens to be one of the best hospitals in the world. A hospital so renowned that my French doctor advised me to remain in the United States to seek treatment rather than return to France. What are the odds that my new job would be located next to this hospital?

But it doesn't end there.

When I called Johns Hopkins to schedule an appointment with a breast cancer surgeon, only the director was available to see me. When I called to schedule my appointment with a new oncologist, only the director was free to see me! I could have had anyone, any doctor, but no one else was available.

I still can't get over it.

All these tiny seemingly coincidences were, in fact, God working behind the scenes, fighting for me. "Wondering why I did not die? God favored me." Yes, Hezekiah. YES!

He saved me.

When I was at my lowest, he sent angels to lift me up. When I was first diagnosed, I called my best friend from Alabama. We were schoolmates. We have been friends since we were six years old. When we were 18, she was saved with such a ferocity that I liken it to Moses at the burning bush. And since age 18 she has been singing and praying and witnessing for God.

Therefore, it was only natural that I reached out to her. In turn, she reached out to other prayer warriors who formed a solid circle of love around me. I felt their prayers from all around the nation, joined with those from around the world. Once when I was talking to my friend, I told her that I wanted to be saved with the same fire that saved and consumed her. She said that I could be. That I should be. That I am. That the same love and strength burns in me as well. And so, after many years of not falling to my knees, I did just that. I prayed with all my heart and soul and mind that God would save me from this terrible disease. I didn't want to die. I wanted to see my children grow up. After all, my youngest was only one year old when I was diagnosed. A baby! There was no way I wanted to or planned to leave her. I asked God to give me the strength I would need to fight this cancer battle. And He did.

There's a military expression that goes like this: "There are no atheists in foxholes." Well, I can tell you, fighting cancer is a foxhole and I haven't run into too many atheists along my journey. Oh, I'm sure they exist, but I haven't met any myself. You might not believe in the God that I believe in and worship. But whatever the case, don't be afraid to allow your spirituality to help you during these challenging days.

Chapter 15
Bible Verses to Help You Along the Way

Psalms 27 is one of my favorite chapters for a reminder of this. When you wake up every day, recite the first verse—even if you cannot recite the entire chapter:

The LORD is my light and my salvation—
whom shall I fear?
The LORD is the stronghold of my life—
of whom shall I be afraid?
2 When the wicked advance against me
to devour me,
it is my enemies and my foes
who will stumble and fall.
3 Though an army besiege me,
my heart will not fear;
though war break out against me,
even then I will be confident.
4 One thing I ask from the LORD,
this only do I seek:
that I may dwell in the house of the LORD
all the days of my life,
to gaze on the beauty of the LORD
and to seek him in his temple.
5 For in the day of trouble
he will keep me safe in his dwelling;

he will hide me in the shelter of his sacred tent
and set me high upon a rock.
6 Then my head will be exalted
above the enemies who surround me;
at his sacred tent I will sacrifice with shouts of joy;
I will sing and make music to the LORD.
7 Hear my voice when I call, LORD;
be merciful to me and answer me.
8 My heart says of you, "Seek his face!"
Your face, LORD, I will seek.
9 Do not hide your face from me,
do not turn your servant away in anger;
you have been my helper.
Do not reject me or forsake me,
God my Savior.
10 Though my father and mother forsake me,
the LORD will receive me.
11 Teach me your way, LORD;
lead me in a straight path
because of my oppressors.
12 Do not turn me over to the desire of my foes,
for false witnesses rise up against me,
spouting malicious accusations.
13 I remain confident of this:
I will see the goodness of the LORD
in the land of the living.
14 Wait for the LORD;
be strong and take heart
and wait for the LORD.

10 Bible verses that Helped Me with Bad News

1. Therefore, we do not lose heart. Though outwardly we are wasting away, yet inwardly we are being renewed day by day. For our light and momentary troubles are achieving for us an eternal glory that far outweighs them all. So we fix our eyes not on what is seen, but on what is unseen, since what is seen is temporary, but what is unseen is eternal. **2 Corinthians 4:16-19**
2. He sent out his word and healed them; he rescued them from the grave. **Psalms 107:20**
3. But those who hope in the LORD will renew their strength. They will soar on wings like eagles; they will run and not grow weary, they will walk and not be faint. **Isaiah 40:31**
4. Be strong and courageous. Do not be afraid or terrified because of them, for the LORD your God goes with you; he will never leave you nor forsake you." **Deuteronomy 31:6**
5. The Spirit himself testifies with our spirit that we are God's children. Now if we are children, then we are heirs—heirs of God and co-heirs with Christ, if indeed we share in his sufferings in order that we may also share in his glory. **Romans 8:16-17**
6. In my distress I called to the LORD; I cried to my God for help. From his temple he heard my voice; my cry came before him, into his ears. **Psalms 18:6**
7. There is a time for everything, and a season for every activity under the heavens: **Ecclesiastes 3:1**
8. Come to me, all you who are weary and burdened, and I will give you rest. Take my yoke upon you and learn from me, for I

am gentle and humble in heart, and you will find rest for your souls. **Matthew 11:28-29**

9. For I know the plans I have for you," declares the LORD, "plans to prosper you and not to harm you, plans to give you hope and a future. **Jeremiah 29:11**
10. "Do not let your hearts be troubled. You believe in God; believe also in me.
    My Father's house has many rooms; if that were not so, would I have told you that I am going there to prepare a place for you? And if I go and prepare a place for you, I will come back and take you to be with me that you also may be where I am. You know the way to the place where I am going." **John 14:1-4**

10 Bible Verses that Helped Me with Faith

1. Now faith is confidence in what we hope for and assurance about what we do not see. **Hebrews 11:1**
2. He says, "Be still, and know that I am God; I will be exalted among the nations, I will be exalted in the earth." **Psalms 46:10**
3. Whoever believes in me, as Scripture has said, rivers of living water will flow from within them. **John 7:38**
4. Consequently, faith comes from hearing the message, and the message is heard through the word about Christ. **Romans 10:17**
5. Overhearing what they said, Jesus told him, "Don't be afraid; just believe." **Mark 5:36**
6. For we live by faith, not by sight. **2 Corinthians 5:7**
7. "Have faith in God," Jesus answered them. Truly, I tell you, if anyone says to this mountain, 'Go, throw yourself into the sea,' and does not doubt in their heart but believes that what they

say will happen, it will be done for them. Therefore I tell you, whatever you ask in prayer, believe that you have received it, and it will be yours. **Mark 11:22-24**

8. So that your faith might not rest on human wisdom, but on God's power. **1 Corinthians 2:5**
9. If you believe, you will receive whatever you ask for in prayer. **Matthew 21:22**
10. For no word from God will ever fail. **Luke 1:37**

10 Bible Verses that Helped Me Deal with Friendships

1. Greater love hath no man than this: to lay down one's life for one's friends. **John 15:13.**
2. One who has unreliable friends soon comes to ruin, but there is a friend who sticks closer than a brother. **Proverbs 18:24**
3. How good and pleasant it is when God's people live together in unity! **Psalms 133:1**
4. Dear friends, let us love one another, for love comes from God. Everyone who loves has been born of God and knows God.**1 John 4:7**
5. If either of them falls down, one can help the other up. But pity anyone who falls and has no one to help them up. **Ecclesiastes 4:10**
6. And he has given us this command: Anyone who loves God must also love their brother and sister. **1 John 4:21**
7. Two are better than one; because they have a good return for their labor. **Ecclesiastes 4:9**
8. For I long to see you so that I may impart unto you some spiritual gift to make you strong-- that is, that you and I may be mutually encouraged by each other's faith. **Romans 1:11-12**

9. As iron sharpens iron, so one person sharpens another. **Proverbs 27:17**
10. Perfume and incense bring joy to the heart, and the pleasantness of a friend springs from their heartfelt advice. **Proverbs 27:9**

Acknowledgements

Many have stood beside me along this journey. Here are a few I'd like to thank in particular.

Janay Podraza, Dorothy Johnson, Forrest Johnson, Deb Heard and Junko Hurley went to Chemotherapy with me. Sherri Chatman told me to "just keep it moving" upon diagnosis, therefore helping me to get out of bed. Paula Robinson Cooley prayed her heart out for me; I thank you.

My Paris family—Arlette and Yann Lalisse, Kim Petyt, Kim Powell, Monique Wells, Frederique Itier, Stephanie Bombrun, Octavie Chakoute, Christelle Hyenne, Mark Clement and the Mark Clement Salon, Bruno Sene, Joëlle Bollanga, Esther Hautebas, Mickael Enkiri, Ayd Adam, and all my former colleagues at ORSYP.

My American family—Rebecca Tsafos, Natalie Lobus, Derek Jones, Tracey Smith, Victor Hamilton, Larry Mack, Pearl Beach, Ronald Bledsoe, Veronica Contreras, Laveechia Wilson, Ida Serrano, Mary Danhires, Hae-Jin Kwon, Kathy Lesnick, John Roy, Ron Snider, Luis Carerro, Millie Hernandez Rothwell, Alberto Bernaola, Katie Park, Alfredo Navarro, Ernest Dixon, Omyra Batiste, Renee Dodd, and Katrina Slaughter Johnson.

To my sister survivors—Kathleen Major, Lise de Lise, Catherine Hargrove, and Joyce Hampton: you are an inspiration.

My amazing fellow editors and writers who worked on this—Deb Heard, Carolyn Moncel, Patrice Gaines, Nicole Shawan Junior, LaTasha James, Sayyah Israel, Beverly East, Gay Byron, Thera Martin, Bill Brantley, Janice Delaney and Rachel Fogg.

And finally, thanks to my outstanding medical team, especially Drs. Fetting, Habibi, Hsu, Cooney, Russell, Asrari, Kayat and Provoust. To Cathi Klein, Marshalee George, Nelli Zafman, Heather Prender, Kathryn McGinty and all the nurses and staff (Jane, Amber, Dawn, Christy)—I will be eternally grateful. A special note of appreciation to my chemotherapy team, Fannie, Jean, Linda and Debbie. You will always hold a special place in my heart.

If I've forgotten anyone, please forgive me and know that I will always be grateful to every single person who has helped me in this fight.

About the Author

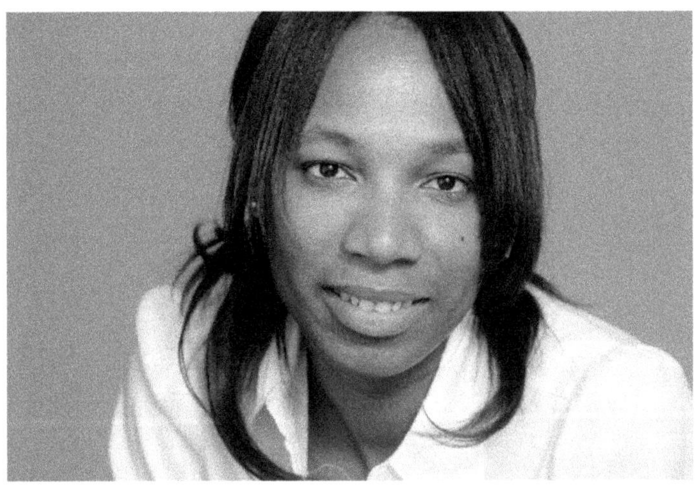

PRISCILLA LALISSE-JESPERSEN, a.k.a. "Prissy," was born and raised in Alabama. Priscilla lived in New York City and worked as an editor, before relocating to Paris.

In 2005, Priscilla published her first novel, *Stockdale*, which takes readers into the small-town life of Cassie Taylor. In 2011, Priscilla published *Next of Kin*, a memoir about losing her father to cancer while living thousands of miles away in France.

Priscilla has contributed to such online publications as Paris Woman Journal, Bonjour Paris, Café de la Soul, Black Entertainment Television and Entrée to Black Paris, where her very personal articles often chronicle the French experience through American eyes. In 2007, she launched her own web magazine, Prissy Mag, which gives readers a unique view into everyday life in Paris, as told by Anglophones who live it.

She has often been featured in the media, including BBC London Radio, Voice of America News, and Entrée to Black Paris, Black Profiles in Paris, Vingt Paris, Expat Radio, Paris Missives, Paris if you Please, My French Life and The OP Life.

Priscilla has been a freelance writer for *The Washington Post* since 2013 and writes articles on politics, culture and travel.

When not writing, she enjoys travelling, learning new languages, and collecting and reading books.

Visit priscilla-lalisse-jespersen.com for more information.

www.ingramcontent.com/pod-product-compliance
Ingram Content Group UK Ltd.
Pitfield, Milton Keynes, MK11 3LW, UK
UKHW022011190726
13853UKWH00004B/1883